MW01227956

African American Health
Peeling Back the Layers for a Vision of the Future

First printing July 2023

Library of Congress Cataloging-in-Publication Data
Lawson, William
african american health: peeling back the layers for a vision of the future / by william lawson, MD, PhD

ISBN: 9798853540538

Published by AR PRESS, an American Real Publishing Company

Roger L. Brooks, Publisher
roger@incubatemedia.us
americanrealpublishing.com
Printed in the U.S.A.

PEELING BACK THE LAYERS FOR A VISION OF THE FUTURE

AFRICAN AMERICAN
HEALTH

LAWSON EDITORIALS

WILLIAM B. LAWSON, MD, PHD

To Robert Lawson and Anthony Lawson, who provided me with a tangible goal for the future.

Contents

About the Articles

These articles are editorials by William B. Lawson MD, PhD when he was Editor in Chief during the 2000s. The journal, at that time, was published by the parent organization, the National Medical Association. Dr. Lawson along with Dr. Chile Ahaghotu MD, MA, EMHL, FAC negotiated with Elsevier, one of the largest academic publishers in the world to become the journal publisher. As a result, the Journal received the financial foundation to continue, and through the added expertise recruited, quality manuscripts continued the mission of the National Medical Association.

Mission of the National Medical Association

The National Medical Association (NMA), as stated on its website, is the collective voice of African American physicians and the leading force for parity and justice in medicine and the elimination of disparities in health.

The NMA is a 501(c)(3) national, professional, and scientific organization representing the interests of more than 50,000 African American physicians and the patients they serve. NMA is committed to improving the quality of health among minorities and disadvantaged people through its membership, professional development, community health education, advocacy, research, and partnerships with federal and private agencies. Throughout its history, the National Medical Association has focused primarily on health issues related to African Americans and medically underserved populations; however, its principles, goals, initiatives, and philosophy encompass all ethnic groups.

History

The National Medical Association in the United States was founded in 1895. It emerged during a time when African American physicians faced significant racial discrimination and exclusion from mainstream medical organizations. The primary motivations for establishing the NMA were:

1. Advocacy: The NMA was created to address the systemic racial discrimination and exclusion that African American physicians experienced in the American Med-

ical Association (AMA) at the time. The AMA, which was the predominant medical association, did not allow African Americans to become members or participate in its activities. The NMA aimed to provide a platform for African American physicians to advocate for their rights and address healthcare disparities affecting African American communities.

2. Professional Development: The NMA sought to promote the professional development and networking opportunities for African American physicians. It aimed to create a supportive environment for African American physicians to collaborate, share knowledge, and enhance their skills. By doing so, the NMA aimed to strengthen the representation and impact of African American physicians within the medical field.

3. Health Equity: The NMA recognized the significant health disparities faced by African American communities due to systemic racism and discrimination. The organization aimed to address these disparities by advocating for policies and initiatives that promote equitable access to healthcare, eliminate racial barriers, and improve the health outcomes of African Americans.

Overall, the National Medical Association was founded to address the exclusion and discrimination faced by African American physicians in mainstream medical organizations, advocate for their rights, promote professional development, and work towards achieving health equity for African American communities.

About the Journal

The JNMA is a peer-reviewed scientific publication that covers a wide range of medical topics, including research articles, clinical studies, public health issues, and health policy. It serves as a platform for healthcare professionals to share their findings and insights with the NMA community and the broader medical field. It has a long and esteemed history within the NMA, which is the oldest and largest organization representing African American physicians and their patients in the United States. The JNMA serves as the official scientific publication of the NMA and covers a wide range of medical topics.

The JNMA was first established in 1909 as the "Journal of the National Medical Association" and has since played a crucial role in disseminating medical knowledge and research within the African American medical community. Over the years, the journal has provided a platform for physicians, researchers, and scholars to publish their findings, share clinical experiences, and discuss important health issues.

The JNMA publishes peer-reviewed articles spanning various disciplines of medicine, including original research, review articles, case reports, and editorials. It cover s topics relevant to the NMA's mission, such as health disparities, community health, cultural competence, an d advancements in medical practice and education.

Throughout its history, the JNMA has been dedicat-ed to advancing medical knowledge, promoting equity in healthcare, and addressing health disparities. It has contributed significantly to the medical literature, high-lighting the achievements and challenges faced by African American physicians and their patients.

Special thanks goes to the Journal of The National Medical Association and Elsevier.

Violence Research

JOURNAL OF THE NATIONAL Medical Association
  Volume 109, Issue 4, Winter 2017, Page 221
  William B. Lawson M.D., Ph.D., D.L.F.A.P.A.
  https://doi.org/10.1016/j.jnma.2017.10.002Get rights and
content

The need for medical knowledge and political expediency has often clashed. Usually, the consequences have limited long-term effects. However, the lack of information can have important consequences for African American providers and patients, who may have disproportionate access to medical services and the newest treatment findings. Recently, a massacre occurred in Las Vegas with over 500 people shot and 58 dead. Much of the debate has focused on whether the perpetrator was mentally ill, if restricting gun access would have prevented such a terrible act, or even whether such acts can be prevented. Examination of motive and data related to a single event will probably not lead to findings that can be generalized for such acts. However, there is very little recent research on gun violence prevention in the United States. Part of the limited research is a result of the belief that such research should be looked at as a criminal justice issue or moral issue and not a public health issue. But, a major factor that limited this research was political.

In 1996, Congress threatened to strip funding from the Centers for Disease Control and Prevention unless it stopped funding research into firearm injuries and deaths because it was thought that such research promoted gun control. As a result, the CDC stopped funding gun-control research. The impact was felt beyond the CDC. The National Institute of Justice, an arm of the U.S. Department of Justice, funded 32 gun-related studies from 1993 to 1999, but none from 2009 to 2012, according to Mayors Against Illegal Guns. The institute then resumed funding in 2013, in the wake of the Sandy Hook Elementary shooting the year before. It's not clear if further research might have produced findings that have prevented this tragedy. The important point is that as gun violence continues to be a major cause of death, especially for African American males, it is one area of public health that has been under-researched. Moreover, there remains a strong belief that such research is politically motivated. The Journal has dedicated this issue, and a subsequent issue, to violence. Hopefully, the publication of such articles will encourage other researchers to develop approaches that can address the prevention and consequences of violence which can have applicability to all medical disciplines.

2

The Need for Basic Science: An Editorial

Journal of the National Medical Association
Volume 109, Issue 2, Summer 2017, Page 69
William B. Lawson M.D., Ph.D., D.L.F.A.P.A.
https://doi.org/10.1016/j.jnma.2017.05.008Get rights and content

Recently, demonstrations were held in Washington DC, not by disgruntled minorities, abortion rights activists, the homeless, or labor protestors, but by scientists, mostly academicians. Their fear is that the change in the federal administration, because of the past election, may be a harbinger of a cutback in governmental support for scientific research. Their concerns have important implications for medical treatment. American medicine is evidence-based, and as much as possible, develops the understanding of disease states from basic science. The irony is that the translation of basic science to medical interventions and improved health care has become faster and more consistent but the impact on the health care of ethnic minorities may now be lessened.

Recognition of ethnic differences in morbidity and mortality are now widely known. African Americans and Latinos consistently show greater disease burden, health care outcomes, and more disease burden in many disease states. The differences are often attributed to socioeconomic status and access to care. But the argument can be made that some of the disparities are a result of a lack of access to the advances seen in medical technology. Often, African Americans are less likely to get access to new treatments which may be more effective or safer. Lack of support for basic research could limit new treatment advances that would be especially more advantageous to ethnic minorities.

Research is in the United States is invariably investigator-initiated. However, minority researchers are rare. All other things being equal, they are less likely to get grant funding. Disease states more common or with worse outcomes in African Americans may be less studied. Ethnic minorities are certainly underrepresented in clinical trials, which could contribute to reducing knowledge gaps in treatment. Limited scientific resources are as important as the increased focus on social equity as contributors to health disparities.

3

The Same Result

JOURNAL OF THE NATIONAL Medical Association
  Volume 111, Issue 1, February 2019, Pages 1-2
  William B. Lawson M.D., Ph.D., D.L.F.A.P.A.
  https://doi.org/10.1016/j.jnma.2019.01.007Get rights and
content

Einstein is widely believed to have said, "The definition
of insanity is doing the same thing over and over but expecting different results." Yet, we have multiple instances
in which we have identified a problem and continue to
watch the problem persist despite ongoing interventions.
Persistence of the problem may be the result of repeating
the same approaches, repackaged, despite the absence of
positive results. Persistence of racial disparities in health
care immediately comes to mind. Such disparities have
been noted since the beginning of medical record doc-
umentation and assessment of public health issues. This
Journal, throughout its history, has documented these dis-

parities. Most importantly, the National Medical Association as one of its primary missions, has continued to make public statements, attempted to develop policies, and promote legislative efforts to change this trajectory.

Articles in this and other issues show, however, that racial disparities in access to care continue to occur. The Journal has done its part in making public the finding of persistence in disparities and some of the efforts to reduce these disparities. Yet, despite the findings, racial disparities in care outcomes continue to persist. Dr. David Satcher, as Surgeon General, consistently documented these disparities and published multiple reports of the disparities, as have others.

In my field of mental health, I noted that African Americans continued to be overdiagnosed with schizophrenia and underdiagnosed with depression or post-traumatic stress disorder despite public awareness campaigns, changes in diagnostic instruments, and extensive published literature.

Why have these various approaches not been successful?

1. Perhaps knowledge based on racist beliefs are not adequately addressed. Studies have shown that medical students and residents continue to harbor face beliefs about race despite their educa-

tion. Current medical education may have to be changed to specifically target misinformation.

2. Perhaps racist attitudes are so pervasive and institutionalized in the system that change is difficult if not impossible. Again, it has been shown that such bias exists among medical students and practitioners.[5] Medical education and continuing medical education may need to directly address such biases. Outside of medicine, changes such as the election of an African American national president, and the election of African American presidents in the American Medical Association show that some change is possible.

3. It may be that we need a diverse workforce to impact all segments of medicine. The percentage of African American male graduates has remained static for half a century. More must be done or different approaches are needed to resolve this all-important disparity.

4. It may be that we still have not found that right program or strategy. There is hope then that we may need to do more, research more, and develop innovative approaches.

5. It may simply be that changes have occurred but

in a way that is too subtle to demonstrate clinically
or there has not been sufficient time to see mean-
ingful results. That would not be heartening to our
patients, but may suggest that we need to do more
to identify approaches that work and disseminate
them. Ultimately, the goal must be to reduce disparities to the extent that there is clinical benefit
to our patients.

Clearly, we as providers, and other stakeholders must
do more. The opportunity is there for new leaders in the
medical community to develop new strategies and approaches. The Journal continues to be receptive to new,
effective approaches and to serve as a means of knowledge dissemination.

References
1Did Einstein really define insanity as doing the same
thing over and over again expecting different results.
https://www.quora.com/Did-Einstein-really-define-ins
anity-as-doing-the-same-thing-over-and-over-again-an
d-expecting-different-results/2018. Accessed 14 January
2018.

2 W.B. Lawson
The one hundredth and tenth anniversary
J Natl Med Assoc, 110 (2018), pp. 529-530,

3 D. Satcher

Eliminating racial and ethnic disparities in health: the role of the ten leading health indicators

J Natl Med Assoc, 92 (2000), pp. 315-318

4M. Gara, W.A. Vega, S. Arndt, *et al.*

Influence of patient race and ethnicity on clinical assessment in patients with affective disorders.

Arch Gen Psychiatr, 69 (2012), pp. 593-600,

5K. Hoffman, S. Trawalter, J. Axta, *et al.*

Racial bias in pain assessment and treatment recommendations, and false beliefs about biological differences between blacks and whites.

Proc Natl Acad Sci, 113 (2016), pp. 4296-4301,

6C. Bright, M. Price, R. Morgan, *et al.*

The report of the W. Montague Cobb/NMA health institute consensus panel on the plight of underrepresented minorities in medical education.

J Natl Med Assoc, 110 (2018), pp. 614-623,

Epub 2018 Jun 5. Review

4

Being an MD is not protective

JOURNAL OF THE NATIONAL Medical Association
Volume 111, Issue 2, April 2019, Page 119
William B. Lawson M.D., Ph.D., D.L.F.A.P.A.
https://doi.org/10.1016/j.jnma.2019.03.002Get rights and content

In recent years, more and more physicians are becoming involved in politics and running for national office. Many of us naively assumed that this would be a good thing. Physicians are trained to care for others, to take an oath of service, and to sacrifice their time and personal needs for their patients. It would seem that physician politicians would be especially concerned about the common good and put issues such as power and political expediency in the background in order to serve their constituents. For those reasons as well as others, many of us were pleased to see a physician become a governor of Virginia. But that experience re-reminded us of another reality. Physicians can hold racist attitudes and beliefs despite their training. Stereotypical beliefs and attitudes do not disappear with a medical education and a commitment to service. The Virginia governor had in his medical yearbook pictures of individuals in blackface and Klans robes. Whether he was one of the individuals in the picture is irrelevant. It was his yearbook. He is considered a liberal so political persuasion unfortunately is not protective from tolerating racist displays. The yearbook was over 20 years old. Yet the medical school did not take action until recently to address such displays. Unfortunately, such events are not unique. One remembers the African American UCLA medical school faculty member, Christian Head who ended up filing a lawsuit after being depicted as a gorilla. The latter was malicious. The former is far more dangerous because it was perceived as benign and had been largely disregarded for over a decade.

It again is well worth reflecting on the efforts of medical education, national organizations, and community organizations over the past decades. African American males have not appreciatively increased in medical school classes. Racial disparities in care still persist. A study of medical students at the University of Virginia showed that myths about African Americans remain a part of their belief system. The experience of the Virginia governor provides a partial answer. Despite public campaigns and statements, despite cultural awareness programs, race and racism continue to be dominant belief systems in our culture for the majority population. It remains such a pervasive belief system that it is taken for granted, to be addressed only when the victims complain.

The challenge for the National Medical Association remains. It must continue to advocate for our patients. It must be unrelenting in confronting racism in the medical profession. It must not stop expecting that all physicians must provide quality care to their patients regardless of race or ethnicity. Most importantly, it must remind our members in training and early career physicians that the need to reduce racial disparities in care remains. Racism in the United States is not ancient history, it continues to be an ongoing reality that will not disappear of its own accord.

References
1B. Tarrant
Virginia Governor Apologizes for Racist Photo but Resists Growing Calls to Quit.
https://www.reuters.com/article/us-virginia-politics-id USKCN1PR001/, Accessed 28th Feb 2019
2 G. Demby

Christian Head, Black UCLA Medical School Doctor, Files Lawsuit After Alleged Gorilla Depiction (2012) , Accessed 28th Feb 2019

3. C.M. Bright, M.A. Price, R.C. Morgan Jr., R.K. Bailey

The report of the W. Montague cobb/NMA health institute consensus panel on the plight of underrepresented minorities in medical education J Natl Med Assoc, 110 (6) (2018 Dec), pp. 614-623,

Epub 2018 Jun 5. Review

4Kelly M. Hoffman, Sophie Trawalter, Jordan R. Axta,

M. Norman Oliver

Racial bias in pain assessment and treatment recommendations, and false beliefs about biological differences between blacks and whites Proc Natl Acad Sci, 113 (2016), pp. 4296-4301,

5

Disparities, Fake News, or Just not the Whole Story

JOURNAL OF THE NATIONAL Medical Association
Volume 110, Issue 4, August 2018, Page 303
William B. Lawson M.D., Ph.D., D.L.F.A.P.A.
https://doi.org/10.1016/j.jnma.2018.07.003Get rights and content

Recently a paper, "Age-Related Racial Disparity in Suicide Rates Among U.S. Youths From 2001 Through 2015" garnered a good deal of national attention. It reported that suicide rates increased from 1993 to 1997 and 2008 to 2012 among black children aged 5–11 years and decreased among white children of the same age, which on the face of it was a shocking finding. Historically, suicide was thought to be rare to nonexistent in African Americans. Reports that suicide rates in African American youth now approach the rates of whites have generated a great deal of distress. In the past, the narrative was that African Americans simply did not get depressed or lacked the mental apparatus to appreciate depression and suicide. More recently the thought was that African Americans were thought to be resilient despite the social, economic, and personal hardships that people of color faced and therefore that these hardships were not that impactful. However, an increasing suicide rate seemed more consistent with other findings that the negative social determinants of health impact not only physical health but mental health. The evidence that suicide rates may be higher in African American children certainly seems to demand a call for action. However, Dr. Carl Bell, an associate editor of the Journal has provided a more measured interpretation. He noted that there were multiple methodological issues that made the conclusion of the article questionable. Because of the small numbers involved, the differences may not be significant. But he raised another issue. Must there be significant disparities in health outcomes to generate the mobilization of resources necessary to address the racism of African Americans? The need to show adversity and disparities certainly is one way to justify the need to focus on the real health needs of African Americans. However, even if racial differences are not present, the importance of addressing problems in the

Black community such as suicide remains. There should be no need to depend as Dr. Bell noted on "fact news."

Interpretation of disparities also has influenced the narrative of opiate-related deaths. The dramatic increase in whites has galvanized the allocation of resources to prevention and treatment for white males. Yet, substance abuse remains a problem in black communities. Moreover, there has been a qualitative difference in approaches. A recent study showed that cocaine-related overdose deaths among non-Hispanic blacks are on par with overdose deaths caused by heroin and prescription opioids among whites. Yet, there has not been an appreciation of the large increase in opioid deaths among African Americans or the focus on punishment and incarceration rather than treatment. Disparities in care should not be the only criteria for focusing on the needs of African Americans. A future issue of the Journal will be devoted to opiate and substance abuse in African Americans, which can be an opportunity to continue this dialogue.

References
1J. Bridge, L. Horowitz, C. Fontanella, *et al.*
Age-related racial disparity in suicide rates among US youths from 2001 through 2015
JAMA Pediatr, 172 (7) (2018), pp. 697-699
2A. Poussaint, Alexander

Lay my burden down: suicide and the mental health crisis among African-Americans revised edition

Beacon Press, Boston (2000)

3 C. Bell

Commentary: Is the Suicide Story Fake- or Just Misleading?

Clinical Psychiatry News (June 14, 2018)

https://www.mdedge.com/psychiatry/article/168142/depression/suicide-story-fake-or-just-misleading

4M. Shiels, N. Freedman, D. Thomas, *et al.*

Trends in U.S. drug overdose deaths in non-hispanic black, hispanic, and non-hispanic white persons, 2000–2015

Ann Intern Med, 168 (600) (2018), pp. 453-455

5J. Netherland, H. Hansen

White opioids: pharmaceutical race and the war on drugs that wasn't.

Biosocieties, 12 (2) (2017), pp. 217-238

6

The Need for Leaders

JOURNAL OF THE NATIONAL Medical Association
Volume 110, Issue 3, June 2018, Page 203
William B. Lawson MD, PhD, DLFAPA,PA, Silver Spring MD
https://doi.org/10.1016/j.jnma.2018.05.001Get rights and content

Soon, an African American, Altha Stewart, will become the president-elect of another major professional medical association, the American Psychiatric Association. At this point, most medical societies have elected at least one African American leader. However, few organizations have elected more than one. Unfortunately, that observation is consistent with the issue of the presence of African Americans in medicine. Despite multiple programs and initiatives, the number of African Americans and African American males, in particular, remain little different from twenty years ago. The aging of current African American providers and the limited number in the pipeline does not bode well for the future of diversity in medicine. Ethnic matching and increasing diversity have been proposed as solutions to the persisting disparities in care that African Americans face. Unfortunately, this strategy will not be practical for the foreseeable future. The issue is not simply the availability of personnel but the importance of leadership. Racial disparities in health delivery systems still persist. Clinical research continues to have limited diversity in investigators and subjects. Fallacies about race are still held among medical students. Increasing leadership diversity may have an impact well before a diverse workforce can be attained.

7

Visiting Black Patients: Racial Disparities in Security Standby Requests

JOURNAL OF THE NATIONAL Medical Association
Volume 110, Issue 2, April 2018, Page 103
William B. Lawson M.D., Ph.D., D.L.F.A.P.A.
https://doi.org/10.1016/j.jnma.2018.03.001Get rights and content

Racial and ethnic disparities in care have been described in the past decade and are consistent with persisting prejudicial behavior and frank racism seen in much of American society. More disturbing is the increasing evidence that such behavior impacts more than quality of life. It can have life and death implications. The most explicit examples are shown in the previous and current issues. The authors consistently make the case that violence is an important public health issue in the African American community. Moreover the killing of unarmed Black men, women, and children by police and security officers are at least in part related to the perception of people of color in this country and not simply a result of socioeconomic factors."

Prejudicial behavior also impacts elements of health care from simple delivery of services. A paper in this issue by Dr. Green and associates reminds us that addressing racial disparities must take into account all aspects of the health delivery system including visitor waiting areas. She and her colleagues noted that African American patients and their visitors were far more likely to generate security standby requests. Specifically, hospital security was called more often for Black patients and their visitors than Whites. The authors note the implications for healthcare disparities, low patient satisfaction, and diminished health outcomes.

Clearly, social determinants of health and structural inequalities must be addressed and dealt with if disparities in care are to be addressed. However, continued observations show that these issues cannot be addressed simply by policy changes, economic improvements, or improving access.

References

1 Institute of Medicine

B.D. Smedley, A.Y. Stith, A.R. Nelson (Eds.), Unequal Treatment: Confronting Racial and Ethnic Am J Public Health, vol. 106 (2016), pp. 2219-2226

1. E. Frazer, R. Mitchell, L. Nesbitt, M. Williams, D. Browne

The violence epidemic in the African American community: a call by the national medical association for com-prehensive reform.

J Natl Med Assoc, 110 (2018), pp. 4-15

3J. Bosman, E.G. Fitzsimmons

Grief and Protests Follow Shooting of a Teenager. Police Say Mike Brown Was Killed after Struggle for Gun in St. Louis Suburb.

The New York Times (2014, August 10)

Retrieved from:

4S. Dewan, R.A. Oppel (Eds.), Tamir Rice Case, Many Errors by Cleveland Police, then a Fatal One, The New York Times (2015 January 22)

Retrieved from:

5Carmen R. Green, Wayne R. McCullough, Jamie D. Hawley, M. Div Visiting black patients: racial disparities in security standby requests.

J Natl Med Assoc (2018), pp. 37-43

8

What is Health Equity?

JOURNAL OF THE NATIONAL Medical Association
  Volume 110, Issue 1, February 2018, Page 1
  William B. Lawson M.D., Ph.D., DLFAPA
  https://doi.org/10.1016/j.jnma.2018.01.004Get rights and
content

The ongoing recognition of disparities in care, especially for people of color, has led to efforts to develop programs and service delivery systems with the stated goal of
health equity. Health equity refers to the study and causes
of differences in the quality of health across different populations. Health equity is different from health equality, as
it refers only to the absence of disparities in controllable
or remediable aspects of health. Recent developments
have shown that social determinants of health are major
factors for people of color. Moreover, poor health itself
has a substantial economic impact. The good news is that
many of the factors that contribute to racial differences in

outcome are related to remediating and modifying social factors that impact access to care. An underlying assumption however is that differences in health outcomes reflect negative life circumstances. Conversely, the implication is that when there are no racial differences, then the goal of equity has been achieved.

However, there are numerous exceptions that require a close examination of the concept of equity. The role of cigarette smoking in negative health outcomes is well-established. Yet African Americans usually smoke fewer cigarettes and start smoking cigarettes at an older age. But isn't the goal of many programs to reduce disparities in African Americans? Has health equity been achieved and surpassed? Unfortunately, not. African Americans are more likely to die from smoking-related diseases than their white counterparts. Moreover, smoking intervention programs target adolescents but for African Americans, the risky population is adults.

Unfortunately, programs and policies that fail to recognize the specific needs of African Americans are all too common. The simplistic assumption that people of color are ok as long as they match their white counterparts can be shortsighted and even dangerous. Moreover, the focus on racial equity can lead to an important missed opportunity. What if there are components in African American culture and lifestyle that lead to the achievement of better health outcomes for everyone?

9

Editors Note Focusing on Violence in the African American Community

JOURNAL OF THE NATIONAL Medical Association
   Volume 109, Issue 3, Autumn 2017, Page 149
   William B. Lawson M.D., Ph.D., D.L.F.A.P.A.
   https://doi.org/10.1016/j.jnma.2017.08.008Get rights and
content

The next issue of the Journal will be the first of several that will have a focus on violence. Violence in multiple ways, contributes to the poorer quality of life seen in the African American community. Homicide continues to be a major cause of death for African Americans. Suicide, which was once thought to be rare in our community, is now recognized as a major contributor to mortality in

young African American men. Moreover, they dispropor-
tionately face violent injury. Spousal abuse and elderly
abuse continue to be unacceptably high in our community. The observation of violence has been associated
with psychopathology and in poor outcomes for youth.
It is a contributor to our community's ability to improve
education, economics, housing, and health care. Despite
multiple efforts to classify violence as a public health
issue, it continues to be regarded by political leaders as a
criminal justice issue. Evidence-based and health-based
policies such as handgun restrictions, treatment for mental and substance abuse disorders, and various attempts to
improve social equity face strong resistance. The articles
in these issues will address policy, health consequences,
and social implications of violence in order to inform
practitioners about the extent and relevance of this problem. Hopefully, policy leaders and practitioners will be
reminded that violence to African Americans can be re-
duced or prevented by public health approaches. Such a
focus may lead to workable solutions that will persist.

References
1E.B. Pathak
Mortality among black men in the USA
J Racial Ethnic Health Disparities (2017)
In press

2J.B. Richardson, C. St Vil, T. Sharpe, M. Wagner, C. Cooper

Risk factors for recurrent violent injury among black men.

J Surg Res, 204 (1) (2016), pp. 261-266

3J.K. Stockman, M.B. Lucea, R. Bolyard, *et al.*

Intimate partner violence among African American and African Caribbean women: prevalence, risk factors, and the influence of cultural attitudes.

Glob Health Action, 7 (2014), p. 24772

4M. DeLisi, J. Alcala, A. Kusiw, *et al.*

Adverse childhood experiences, commitment offense, and race/ethnicity: are the effects crime-, race-, and ethnicity-specific?

Int J Environ Res Public Health, 14 (3) (2017)

10

Politics and science

JOURNAL OF THE NATIONAL Medical Association
Volume 108, Issue 3, Autumn 2016, Page 137
William B. Lawson M.D., Ph.D., DLFAPA
https://doi.org/10.1016/j.jnma.2016.07.004Get rights and content

Over the past year, we have witnessed numerous tragedies—the murder of mainly LGBT men and women, the deaths of Alton Sterling, Philando Castile, and five police officers in Dallas and three in Baton Rouge. In addition, there were devastating incidents in Charleston, San Bernadino, and Ferguson, and here in Austin—the shooting death of an African American teenager, David Joseph. These tragedies have been presented as evidence that our nation, social fiber, race relations, and governance are falling apart. However, the data shows otherwise. Violent crimes are down, and violence-related deaths are actually fewer than at the beginning of the decade. Nevertheless, they highlight the continued legacy of racism and disparities in political power, socioeconomic status, and access to resources. Solutions to these problems cannot simply come from national leadership and politicians but must include our local communities and national organizations of color. Politicians must have factual information and access to problem-solving technologies. By virtue of their role, physicians often are in the best position to provide local leadership or to be the reservoirs of information.

Physicians, by inclination and training, are healers first and provide a unique perspective when other institutions only offer punitive solutions. These problems often cut across disciplines as they are affected by attempts to deal with lack of services, attempts to self-medicate stress and chronic pain, and the ongoing challenges of functioning in communities that make daily life a chore, especially when chronic illnesses go untreated due to a lack of access to services or resources.

As a national organization of health providers, we must continue to provide a voice for those who are often unable to, to offer solutions based on support rather than punishment, and to provide our patients and local community answers to questions based on facts, rather than prejudice. In these difficult times, we need to support our communities, provide the knowledge base that may lead to workable solutions, and lead the development of policies that will improve the quality of life for our communities. This journal will continue to play a role in building on the foundation of knowledge that will lead to better treatments of our patients. It will provide a peer-driven foundation for the development of effective policies that can lead to sustainable solutions.

11

Editor's Note

JOURNAL OF THE NATIONAL Medical Association
   Volume 108, Issue 2, Summer 2016, Page 103
   William B. Lawson M.D., Ph.D., DLFAPA
   https://doi.org/10.1016/j.jnma.2016.05.004Get   rights
and content

Recently, a widely reported study of medical students at a prestigious university showed that many of them had numerous false beliefs about African Americans, including beliefs that people of color are less sensitive to pain and had thicker skin. Such beliefs unfortunately are probably not isolated and may be widely held by practitioners. They contribute to the mounting evidence previously documented in this Journal that altitudinal factors in the larger society are a factor in racial differences in health outcomes. Focusing on economic disparities and access to insurance, while important, is not enough. Neither is simply geographically improving access to care centers.

Inferior care will be provided as long as the providers continue to hold nonscientific beliefs about the physiology of people of color. Such findings show the importance of organizations such as the National Medical Association which has been outspoken in the need to address racial bias. It also emphasizes the importance of involving the voice of the NMA and its membership in medical education. There simply are not enough providers of color to address the health needs of African Americans so ethnic matching is not a practical solution. More clearly needs to be done to ensure that quality care is received regardless of the ethnicity of the provider.

Reference

1Kelly. Hoffman, Sophie Trawalter, Jordan R. Axt, M. Norman Oliver

Racial bias in pain assessment and treatment recommendations, and false beliefs about biological differences between blacks and whites

Proc Natl Acad Sci, 113 (2016), pp. 4296-4301,

http://www.pnas.org/content/113/16/4296.abstract?tab=author-info-aff-1

About the Author

William B. Lawson, M.D., Ph.D., D.L F.A.P.A.

Dr. Lawson is Founder and Director of the Institute for Reducing Disparities, LLC, President of Senior Psychiatrists Inc, Director of Psychiatric Research for the Emerson Clinical Research Institute, Professor of Psychi-atry and Behavioral Sciences at the George Washington University and the University of Maryland School of Med-icine. He is emeritus professor of psychiatry, at the Dell Medical School, University of Texas, Austin, and emeritus professor and former chair of psychiatry and behavioral sciences at Howard University School of Medicine.

He received a Ph.D. in Psychology from the University of New Hampshire and MD from the Pritzker School of Medicine University of Chicago, did his residency at Stanford University, and a fellowship at the National Institute of Mental Health. He has held faculty positions at the University of Illinois, Urbana, University of California, Irvine, Vanderbilt University, University of Arkansas, and Howard University. He has held numerous senior positions and received national recognition including past President of the DC chapter of Mental Health America,. past president of the Washington Psychiatric Society, past Chair of the Section of Psychiatry and Behavioral Sciences of the National Medical Association, and past president of the Black Psychiatrists of America.

He received the American Psychiatric Foundation Award for Advancing Minority Mental Health, the Solomon Carter Fuller Award by the American Psychiatric Association, the Sigma XI the scientific honor society and Alpha Omega Alpha, the medical honor society, the National Alliance for the Mentally Ill Exemplary Psychiatrist Award and Outstanding Psychologist Award, the Jeanne Spurlock Award from the American Psychiatric Association, the E.Y. Williams Clinical Scholar of Distinction Award from the NMA, and the George Winokur Clinical Research Award from the American Academy of Clinical Psychiatrists. He has over 200 publications and is a former editor-in-chief of the Journal of the National Medical Association. He has continuously received federal, industry, and foundation funding to address mental and substance abuse disparities. He currently serves as the President of Senior Psychiatrists, Inc.

Made in the USA
Columbia, SC
24 January 2025

52425066R00033